LOW-IMPACT
AEROBICS

Other books by Kathryn Lance

Running for Health and Beauty

Getting Strong

A Woman's Guide to Spectator Sports

Total Sexual Fitness for Women

Sportsbeauty

KATHRYN LANCE

LOW-IMPACT AEROBICS

WITH PHOTOGRAPHS BY JILL LEVINE

CROWN PUBLISHERS, INC., NEW YORK

Publisher's Note:
This book contains exercise instructions to be
followed within the context of a complete exercise
program. However, not all exercises are designed for all
individuals. Before starting these or any other exercises
or exercise programs a physician should be consulted.
The instructions in this work are not intended as a
substitute for professional medical advice.

Published by Crown Publishers, Inc.,
225 Park Avenue South, New York, New York 10003
and represented in Canada by
the Canadian MANDA Group

CROWN is a trademark of Crown Publishers, Inc.

Manufactured in the United States of America

Library of Congress Cataloging-in-Publication Data

Lance, Kathryn.
  Low-impact aerobics.

  1. Exercise. I. Title.
GV481.L33   1988   613.7'1   87-22268

ISBN 0-517-56716-4

10 9 8 7 6 5 4 3 2 1

First Edition

CONTENTS

AMERICA GOES AEROBIC

Since the early seventies, the United States has seen a fitness boom that has sent millions to swimming pools, bike paths, tennis courts, and jogging trails. Health-club memberships have soared, as have sales of brightly colored warmup suits, leg-warmers, stretch tights, and "aerobic shoes."

Has all this activity resulted in a healthier America? In part, yes. According to a recent Gallup Poll, approximately 50 percent of all Americans report that they work out regularly, as opposed to 24 percent in 1961. But exercise experts estimate that only 12 to 15 percent of adult Americans are getting enough of the right kind of exercise.

Those Americans who are active give a variety

of reasons for participating in an exercise regimen: to lose weight, relax, improve coordination. But the most important reason for exercise is often overlooked—the need to exercise the most important muscle in the body, the heart. And for this, only aerobic exercise is effective.

What Is Aerobics?

To many Americans, "aerobics" means one thing: aerobic dance. This tremendously popular workout combines dance steps with vigorous jumping and calisthenics. So strong is the public's perception of a connection between aerobic dance and the word aerobics that entire lines of athletic equipment, including shoes, are marketed for "aerobics"—i.e., aerobic dance.

However, the truth is that aerobic dance is only one of many forms of aerobic exercise. Others include jogging, walking, cycling, and swimming. The one thing that all of these exercises have in common is that they promote cardiovascular fitness—fitness of the heart, lungs, and circulatory system.

How aerobic exercises do this is hinted at by the very name aerobics, whose roots come from the Greek words meaning oxygen and life. You can live without food for weeks and water for days, but you cannot go without oxygen for more than a very few minutes. This is because oxygen is required for all processes of life that consume energy, from playing tennis to digesting a meal.

When you do not get a sufficient supply of oxygen, your body lets you know immediately, with pain, fatigue, and shortness of breath. You have probably experienced this "oxygen debt" when running for a bus or after climbing several flights of stairs: your heart pounds and you gasp for breath as your body tries desperately to take in enough oxygen to "pay" for the energy you have expended. Any activity—from running for a bus to doing wind sprints—that puts you into oxygen debt is known as anaerobic, which means "without oxygen."

Aerobic exercises, on the other hand, are those that actually increase your ability to take in and deliver oxygen to all your body tissues. The best aerobic exercises are those in which you breathe deep and hard (but don't gasp) over a sustained period of time, your heart beats faster than usual, and you break out in a sweat.

Some sports, such as tennis, have elements that are both aerobic and anaerobic. However, to positively affect the condition of your cardiovascular system, any aerobic exercise must be performed continuously over a sustained period—twenty minutes is generally recognized as a minimum.

Because of their stop-and-go nature, such vigorous sports as tennis and handball do not provide a sustained aerobic workout.

WHY AEROBIC EXERCISE IS A MUST

All exercise is beneficial; your body is, after all, a machine made for movement. Yet an estimated 40 to 50 percent of all American adults are totally sedentary—and sedentary living is largely responsible for a number of the woes that plague modern Americans, including stiff joints, excessive weight, and osteoporosis. Almost any exercise is better than none, and all forms of exercise have at least some proven benefits. Weight training, for example, will strengthen your muscles and give muscle definition; yoga will improve flexibility; gymnastics can confer grace and coordination. Each of these, and many others, can be part of a varied diet of activity and exercise. However, only aerobic exercise can improve the strength and endurance of your heart. If you only have time for one form of exercise, it should be aerobic.

Aerobic exercise improves your cardiovascular health in a number of ways, but the key to its effectiveness is the sustained period of time spent on the exercise. During this time your heart is forced to work hard, and like any muscle that works hard, it becomes stronger. At the same time, your breathing becomes more efficient as the muscles in your chest grow stronger. There is even some evidence that the capacity of your lungs may increase, allowing them to process greater amounts of oxygen.

As the efficiency of your heart and lungs improves, the resting pulse rate goes down, because your heart has become able to deliver more oxygenated blood with each beat. The result is that you can do more work with less effort. Furthermore, growing evidence indicates that regular aerobic exercise can help prevent and perhaps even reverse atherosclerosis, the progressive clogging of body arteries, which can lead to heart attack and stroke.

All of the health changes discussed so far are profound, and by themselves are reason enough to begin an aerobics program. But the rewards of aerobic exercise go far beyond the immediate cardiovascular benefits and include the following:

● WEIGHT LOSS. Whether you need to lose many pounds or only a few, all studies show that the fastest, most effective way to do so is by combining diet with exercise. First, and most obvious, exercise in itself burns calories. Second, moderate exercise can have an appetite-suppressing effect. And finally, recent studies show that regular exercise speeds up your metabolism—the rate at which you use energy—so that you actually burn more calories all day long and not just when you're working out.

But even if you don't lose much weight, aerobic exercise can help you to look thinner as muscle tissue begins to replace fat. Muscle weighs more than fat but takes up less space, so the net effect is a slimmer, trimmer you. Also, as your muscles become stronger, your posture will improve, resulting in a more youthful, streamlined appearance.

● PROTECTION AGAINST OSTEOPOROSIS. Osteoporosis, or "brittle bones," affects twenty-four million Americans, most of them postmenopausal women. While calcium and estrogen supplementation are commonly used to prevent or treat this crippling condition, new research is focusing on the role of exercise in osteoporosis therapy. Researchers at a recent international conference on osteoporosis recommended three to four hours per week of vigorous exercise for Americans of all ages, explaining that it may increase bone mass at maturity and reduce bone loss later.

● *RELIEF FROM STRESS. Stress, a catchword for the pressures and hassles of a busy life, is thought to be responsible for a variety of ills ranging from depression and insomnia to actual physical illness (stress is believed to weaken the immune system). While anyone under excessive pressure should try to reduce the sources of stress, stress management experts recommend aerobic exercise, among other measures, as an excellent way to help cope. It is believed that exercise somehow increases production of certain brain chemicals that act as the body's own natural tranquilizers. In addition, the physical movement of aerobic exercise can help to relax tense muscles.*

● *IMPROVEMENT OF SELF-IMAGE. Regular aerobic exercise can actually make you look younger, healthier, and more vibrant. In part, this is because of the physical effects we've been talking about—weight loss, improved muscle tone and posture, and better circulation, which can improve skin tone. But exercise also provides a more intangible benefit, one that's especially striking if you've never exercised in your life or have been sedentary for many years—and that is that it actually makes you feel good about yourself. Although you will not notice all of the physical benefits of aerobic exercise right away* (after all, it has taken you years to get out of shape, so it will take weeks or months to regain fitness), most new exercisers notice that they begin to feel better from the very first exercise session. Furthermore, because your stamina and capacity to do aerobic work increase rapidly, the incremental improvements from session to session provide a real incentive to keep going, as well as a feeling that you are accomplishing something. Because of these effects, most first-time exercisers discover a new self-confidence and energy that they have not experienced for years—if ever.

● ENJOYMENT. Finally, aerobic exercise can be fun. It is a break in the day. If you exercise to music, it can feel a lot like dancing. Exercisers can work in groups or pairs, making it a social occasion as well. As hundreds of thousands of aerobics addicts would agree, once you experience the joys of physical movement, you will wonder how you ever did without it.

WHICH AEROBIC EXERCISE IS BEST? 2

No one aerobic exercise is best for everyone. Not only are your age and present physical condition important considerations, but so are your lifestyle and personal preferences. Before taking a closer look at low-impact aerobics, let's briefly examine the most popular aerobic exercises.

WALKING

Walking is so natural that it is strange to think of it as an exercise, but it can be one of the best. Walking becomes aerobic when two conditions are met: when it is done continuously (no stopping to window-shop) and when it is done vigorously enough to raise the heart rate to the training level (see chapter 3). Because walking causes minimal stress to the joints, it is a good beginning aerobic activity, and all that may be needed by elderly exercisers. It should be the foundation for any low-impact program. (For more details, see chapter 4.)

JOGGING

Perhaps the most visible aerobic exercise, jogging for health sparked the fitness boom in the mid-seventies. Jogging is in many ways the most practical and efficient aerobic exercise because it delivers maximum aerobic benefits for a minimal expenditure of time, because it can be done almost anywhere, and because there is nothing to learn and nothing to buy except a pair of jogging shoes.

The main drawback to jogging is that, because of its jarring, high-impact nature, foot, knee, and hip injuries can occur. Injuries are especially likely for "serious runners," those who regularly run more than fifteen miles a week and frequently enter races. Health joggers who run slowly and keep their mileage under fifteen miles per week are less likely to suffer injury. Still, many people find it hard to stick to a jogging program because of boredom or simple dislike of the activity.

Swimming

Another excellent aerobic exercise, swimming delivers all the benefits of aerobics with virtually no danger of injury. Furthermore, swimming tends to condition the entire body, because both the upper and lower body muscles are involved in swimming motions.

The drawbacks to swimming are obvious: it is necessary to know how to swim and to have access to a pool.

Cycling

When it can be performed continuously (in a park, say, rather than in stop-and-go city traffic), cycling is another popular aerobic exercise. Although it is not jarring like jogging, cycling can cause injuries, especially for those who have preexisting hip and knee problems. It is perhaps best for those who have access to a large city park or who live in the country, but it can also be done at home or at a gym on a stationary bike. Cycling is easy and, once you have a bicycle, inexpensive.

AEROBIC DANCE

Aerobic dance was developed by fitness instructor Jackie Sorenson, who noticed that many people failed to stick with an aerobic walking, jogging, or swimming program because it became tedious. She decided to take the boredom out of exercise by making it fun, more like dance, and based her routines on running in place, jumping, lunging, and vigorous dance steps. Combined with driving music and an enthusiastic instructor, aerobic dance seemed more like a social occasion than exercise.

Sorenson's plan was inspired, and aerobic dance and its imitations have become big business across the United States. Aerobic dance continues to enjoy well-deserved popularity, but in the last few years it has become clear that, like jogging, the impact involved in aerobic dance can cause injuries, most often to the ankle, knee, and hip. In fact, one widely publicized survey found that 72 percent of aerobic dance instructors and 44 percent of their students had suffered injuries. This information is misleading, however. According to Dr. Steven Blair of the Institute for Aerobic Research, the studies were flawed scientifically. He feels that more accurate figures for injury, wherein injury is defined as any pain or discomfort that causes the subject to stop the activity for a time, would be 10 percent for instructors and 20 percent for participants. As for injuries severe enough to require medical care, Dr. Blair feels the rate is very small—perhaps as little as one percent. The fact remains, however, that aerobic dance does involve very vigorous movements, including jumping and leaping, which may be difficult or stressful for some people.

Does all this mean, then, that the quest for fitness is doomed to failure because of injury, lack of know-how, or boredom? It was the desire to answer these questions with a resounding no that motivated a number of fitness instructors to develop low-impact aerobics. (These routines are also known by other names, including "minimal-impact" and "no-impact.") The idea behind low-impact aerobics is to avoid jarring and twisting movements, thus reducing the chance of injury or stress.

Low-impact aerobics routines are similar to aerobic dance in that they "look" more like dance than like calisthenics. But in low-impact routines, at least one foot is on the ground at all times, and there are no sudden, violent motions like jumping or lunging. Examples of low-impact aerobics steps are walking in place, high-stepping, and stepping from side to side. In addition to the gentler foot and leg movements, low-impact routines also use the upper body extensively, with the arms remaining at or above shoulder level most of the time.

Can such an exercise regimen be truly aerobic?

The experts are somewhat divided in answer to this. Remember that to be truly aerobic an exercise must fulfill three conditions: it must be continuous, it must be vigorous enough to raise a sweat, and it must raise the exerciser's pulse rate to the training zone (see chapter 3).

Because they involve rhythmic, repetitive movements, low-impact aerobic routines can certainly be performed continuously. And increasing the rate at which each exercise is performed can certainly increase its difficulty and raise the heart rate.

Nevertheless, while low-impact routines may be effective for many people, at least at first, it is doubtful that people who are already fit can obtain a complete aerobic effect from low-impact aerobics alone, and for these people low-impact aerobics should probably be used only as a supplement to another aerobic routine, or as a substitute when recovering from injury.

In fact, combining low-impact aerobics with other routines is good advice for everyone; varying your exercise regimen is the best way to keep it fresh and challenging. The program in this book combines low-impact dance exercises with aerobic walking. The two routines complement each other, because they work the arm and leg muscles in different ways.

WHO CAN DO LOW-IMPACT AEROBICS?

As the preceding discussion should make clear, low-impact aerobics can be done by virtually everyone. Because it puts minimal stress on the joints, it is appropriate for many people who have had injuries or are overweight. And because its intensity can easily be varied by the rate at which the exercises are performed, it is ideal for beginners, the elderly, and anyone who is currently very out of shape. (Although be sure to get your doctor's okay; see following page.)

IMPORTANT NOTE

All exercise and diet books, including this one, warn readers to check with a doctor before beginning a new routine. That warning is included partly to protect the author from lawsuits, but also because it is good advice.

Although some form of exercise is good for nearly everyone, even those with serious medical conditions, unsupervised exercise can be fatal. Many people have heart or artery disease without realizing it, and beginning an aerobics program can cause the condition to grow worse or even precipitate a heart attack.

Even if you think you are as healthy as a horse, please consult with a doctor before starting this or any other program. The necessity of obtaining medical advice is especially important if you are over thirty-five, very overweight, very out of shape, or have a family history of heart disease.

But remember also that once you begin exercising with your doctor's advice, you will become healthier and feel healthier with every day. So turn to the next chapter and we'll get started.

ALL ABOUT EXERCISE

3

If you have never engaged in a regular exercise program in your life, or are starting after several years' layoff, you may be dreading the prospect. Yet the truth is that nothing is easier than starting an exercise program—the trick is sticking with it. One reason so many people drop out of exercise regimens is that they begin with unrealistic expectations, or do not build in incentives to continue. The following discussion may not answer all your questions, but it should help you plan your aerobics program realistically and in a way that will help you incorporate it into your own lifestyle.

WHERE TO DO LOW-IMPACT ROUTINES

For the low-impact aerobic dance routine, the best place to work out is in your own home or that of a neighbor. Most aerobic dance and low-impact classes are given in gymnasiums or dance studios.

The best surface on which to perform the routines is a firm one that is not too hard. A wooden floor is ideal; if your floor is not wood, then you might want to consider exercising on a carpet (but not one that is plush or thick, because some routines involve sliding your foot along the floor). If you are lucky enough to have a backyard patio or terrace, you can perform your activities there and get a little fresh air and sunshine at the same time. Especially when you are first learning the routines, it can be helpful to practice in front of a full-length mirror, and compare your performance to the illustrations in chapter 4.

For suggestions on where to do aerobic walking, see the next chapter.

WHEN TO EXERCISE

You can perform low-impact aerobics at any time of the day or night—whenever is convenient for you. Be certain, though, that you have half an hour or so of uninterrupted time (twenty minutes for the routines, ten minutes for warmup and warmdown). If necessary, take your phone off the hook—remember that the key to achieving aerobic fitness is the continual, uninterrupted nature of the exercise.

Don't exercise within half an hour to an hour of eating—in fact, it is best to wait two hours after a full meal before beginning your routine. This is because your blood supply is devoted to digestion after a meal; if you suddenly begin vigorous exercise, blood must be diverted to your muscles, and this may result in cramps. (This is why you were told as a child never to go swimming within an hour after eating.) Likewise, it is not a good idea to exercise within an hour or two of bedtime—your body needs time to relax after the stimulation of vigorous physical activity.

Bear in mind that low-impact dance aerobics, unlike some other aerobic exercises, can be performed any time of the year and in any weather, because you needn't go outside. If you have an air conditioner, even the dog days of summer won't tempt you to miss a session.

You may enjoy doing your dance routine as a warmup before walking aerobically. In that case, do not exercise too vigorously, and remember to do stretching warmups as well.

WHAT TO WEAR

One of the nicest benefits of the fitness movement has been the proliferation of inexpensive (as well as expensive), attractive, fashionable exercise clothes. Although you can wear anything at all to exercise in, you may enjoy getting one or two brightly colored outfits to "get in the mood." Such clothing can make you feel good about yourself and may serve as an incentive to continue with the program.

Whatever you choose, be it striped leotards and tights or an old gym suit you haven't worn in twenty years, the clothes should be nonbinding and allow full freedom of movement. They should also be lightweight—you will be exercising vigorously and sweating. Likewise, never exercise in rubberized warmup suits, which can cause you to overheat and may even cause heatstroke.

As for accessories, such as leg-warmers, wear whatever makes you feel good. Such fashionable *accessories will make no difference in the performance of your exercises, or even in the amount of time it takes you to warm up.*

It is a good idea to get a good pair of "aerobic" shoes. Although the support provided by such shoes is far more important for high-impact aerobics such as jogging and aerobic dance, the fact is that low-impact routines are performed on your feet, and, especially if you are not used to exercising, the extra support may mean the difference between comfort and sore feet or even injury. You can buy "aerobic" shoes in any sporting goods store or specialty shoe store. Expect to spend at least thirty dollars, but remember that they will last a long time and can double as walking shoes.

EXERCISING TO MUSIC

Although it is not absolutely necessary, most regular exercisers find that exercise time is more enjoyable and that the routines are easier to perform to music (they are, after all, regular, rhythmic steps much like dance). At least one study, in fact, has found that joggers who run while listening to music on headphones achieve a deeper state of relaxation than those who run without music.

When you are first beginning to learn the routines, you may find that music distracts you from concentrating on proper form and on moving smoothly from routine to routine. Once you are familiar with the routines, however, by all means add music. Aerobic dance classes usually rely on music with an insistent beat, such as disco or hard rock. If such music is not to your taste, simply search the radio dial or your own record collection until you find something with a steady, "danceable" beat. If you have a tape recorder and want to take the time, you might try making a twenty-minute tape of some of your favorite tunes.

MAKING IT A PART OF YOUR LIFE

An exercise program is a waste of time if you don't keep it up on a regular basis—a minimum of three times a week, though five times a week is better. But how to keep going? Here are some

*tips that may make it easier for you to make
aerobics truly a part of your life.*

● *SET ASIDE A REGULAR TIME. Make an
appointment with yourself to always exercise at
the same time. This serves two purposes. One is
that the body seems to "get used" to a regular
workout at a regular time and will begin to
respond to it better. The other is that, if you set
aside the time and make certain not to make
other plans for that time, you will be less likely to
make excuses for not working out on days when
you don't feel like it.*

● *FIND A BUDDY. This is one of the best ways
to ensure that you will keep up your program.
Find someone to exercise with, and make a
commitment to work out together three to five
times a week. You can give each other moral
support and also check each other, making sure
you are performing the exercises correctly. You'll
discover that having someone to talk to while
walking will make your exercise time speed by.
And even if you don't feel like exercising on a
given day, you wouldn't want to let down your
buddy, would you?*

● *KEEP A RECORD. This is an almost foolproof*

motivator. Keep a notebook to record your routines and also your goals. After each exercise session, write down what you did during that session. (For example: "Walked one mile in 20 minutes. Felt great!" or "Dance routine twice in 18 minutes.") Just seeing your own progress over a few weeks' time can provide the motivation to continue.

Your own goals will, of course, be as individual as you are. Possibilities include loss of weight, loss of inches, or simply the ability to exercise in your target zone for increasing periods of time until you reach twenty consecutive minutes.

YOUR TARGET HEART RATE

Since the main goal of aerobic exercise is to improve the condition of your heart, it is important to work at a pace that is vigorous enough to challenge your heart but not so vigorous that you become exhausted. That rate is known by a number of different names, including "training rate" and "target heart range" or "zone."

The target heart zone is not a fixed rate (such

as 140 beats per minute) but rather a range. Your own target zone depends to a great extent on your age, but will also very somewhat depending on your present physical condition. When you are exercising in your target zone, your heart will beat noticeably faster than when it is at rest. But it should not beat so fast that you have a feeling of it "thumping" in your chest or you find yourself out of breath. Conversely, if your heart is beating so slowly that you feel you could continue to exercise indefinitely, you probably need to increase the vigor of your workout.

There are a number of formulas for determining your target zone with some accuracy, although such a restricted, "scientific" approach may not be necessary for most people (see below). Still, if you would like to know your own target heart range, make the following calculations:

1. Determine your resting heart rate. This is the number of strokes your heart beats per minute when you have been resting quietly for a while (but not after a meal). The easiest way to take your pulse is to lightly rest two fingertips on the carotid artery in your neck, just below your jaw line. Count your heart beats for fifteen seconds, then multiply by four for your heart rate per minute.

2. Subtract your age from 220.
3. From the result of this subtraction, subtract your resting heart rate.
4. Multiply this new number by .5 and .7.
5. Add your resting heart rate to each new result.

These two new numbers will give you the upper and lower limits of your optimum target heart rate—the zone within which you should aim to work when you are exercising.

Example: For a 43-year-old with a resting heart rate of 67:

1. Resting rate is 67
2. $220 - 43 = 177$
3. $177 - 67 = 110$
4. $.5 \times 110 = 55$
5. $7 \times 110 = 77$
6. $55 + 67 = 122$
7. $77 + 67 = 144$

Thus, this person's target heart range is 122 to 144 beats a minute. Anything over 144 beats would be too vigorous for a maximum training effect, while anything less than 122 would not be strenuous enough to challenge the heart.

When you are first beginning your aerobics program, you may want to stop and check your pulse frequently to be certain that you are not exercising either too strenuously or too easily.

After a while, though, you should develop a "feel" for how vigorously you are working out. In fact, Dr. Steven Blair of the Institute for Aerobics Research feels that there is no need to actually measure your heart rate while you exercise, calling such an approach "too restricted." Rather, he urges, "Start out with what you can do. Walk vigorously. Gradually increase the pace."

This is very good advice and all that is necessary for most people. A good rule of thumb for determining if you are in your target heart range without taking your pulse: if you feel that you are getting a real workout but can still carry on a conversation (or talk to yourself or sing), then you are probably exercising within your target range.

How to Breathe

In some exercise regimens, such as weight training, it is very important to breathe in on certain movements and out on others. In aerobics, such a restricted approach is unnecessary. In both the walking and dance parts of the program, simply breathe naturally, as your body dictates, and don't hold your breath. If you find yourself gasping, you are working out too vigorously and should decrease your pace.

LEARNING THE ROUTINES

In the next chapter you will find guidelines for a two-part low-impact aerobics program: the basic aerobic walking program and a routine of low-impact dance exercises. Included also are warmups and some supplemental and substitute exercises. The dance routine consists of eight exercises, to be performed sequentially. A wide variety of exercises is provided for two reasons: first, the more varied the routines you do, the more muscle groups you exercise; and second, a variety of exercises will help to keep the routine interesting.

However, even though the exercises are easy to do and are presented with photographs and step-by-step instructions, it will still be necessary for you to practice until you can perform them easily without thinking about it. For this reason, it is best to begin your low-impact dance routine by choosing only three or four exercises initially. Walk through each exercise several times until you feel familiar with it. Then try walking through the exercises sequentially. If you are working out in front of a mirror, you might want to tape up a reminder of which routine follows which.

This preparation is necessary not only so you will do the exercises correctly, but also because the key to the aerobic effect is the sustained nature of the exercises. During a workout you must make a transition immediately from one exercise to another, without taking time out to look up how to do the next routine. (If you get confused or lose your place, simply walk briskly in place before going on to the next exercise.)

When you feel you are comfortable with the exercises you have chosen, you can begin to put them together, with music, if you wish. As you become fitter and more adept at the exercises, learn and then add in the others, until your routine consists of eight consecutive exercises. No matter how many separate exercises you do, remember to start out slowly and increase the pace gradually.

For most people, doing the entire sequence of eight exercises should take about five or six minutes. Thus, repeating the sequence three or four times will consume about twenty minutes. If it takes you more or less time to do the routines, adjust by performing more repetitions of some exercises, or by adding or dropping some exercises. Remember that your goal is to work in your target heart zone for twenty consecutive minutes.

THE PROGRAM 4

PART I

AEROBIC WALKING

There is no exercise easier or more natural than walking. All you need to get started is a good pair of walking shoes and a place to walk: a nearby park or schoolyard, a beach, local sidewalks. Bear in mind, however, that it is difficult to walk aerobically on crowded city sidewalks because of congestion and the necessity to stop for traffic lights. If you live in a suburban area, an ideal spot might be a nearby mall. Many malls in all parts of the country are opening their doors early to accommodate aerobic walkers. Because they are covered, these shopping arcades provide perfect indoor tracks for all-weather walking.

As you begin your aerobic walking program, remember the following principles:

● Start out slowly to warm up, then gradually increase the pace.

● Walk continuously, with your heart in its target zone for at least twenty minutes. Allow your arms to pump naturally in rhythm with your steps.

● Walk more slowly to cool down.

When you first begin, limit your walk to five or ten minutes until your stamina improves. Gradually increase your time until you can walk continuously for half an hour (five minutes to warm up, twenty minutes at your target heart rate, and five minutes to cool down). Continue to walk for at least half an hour five or more times a week.

PART II

LOW-IMPACT AEROBIC DANCE ROUTINES

WARMUPS

Although the low-impact dance routines are not particularly strenuous, it is still a good idea to warm up for a few minutes to reduce the chance of injury. After all, you wouldn't expect your car to start right up on a cold day, and neither should you expect your muscles to start with no preparation. Note that many of the warmups are similar to the motions in the dance routines, but are performed less vigorously.

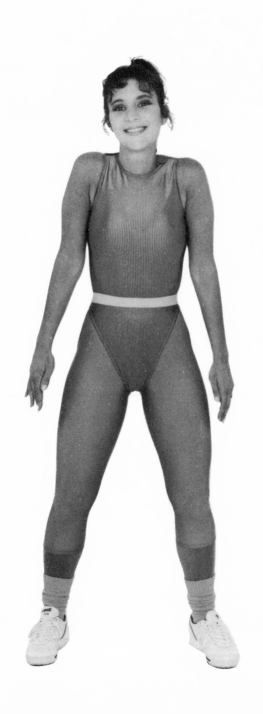

1. Shrug It Off

Stand comfortably with your arms at your sides. Take a deep breath, then, continuing to breathe naturally, begin to make large circles from the front to the back with your shoulders. Exaggerate the motion—imagine that you are trying to touch your ears with the tops of your shoulders. Do four shoulder shrugs from the back to the front, then reverse direction and do four shrugs from the front to the back. Repeat the sequences for a total of sixteen shrugs.

TIP:
_____

Exercise at the same time each day.
Make it a real routine.

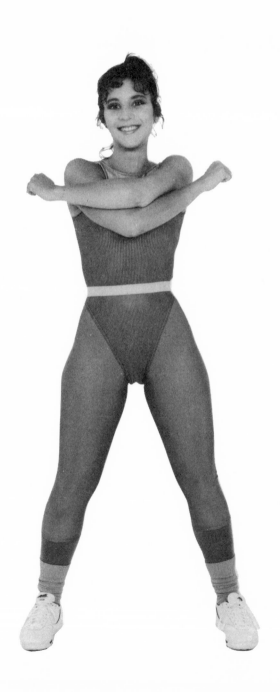

2. Hugs

Stand comfortably with your arms bent slightly above waist level. Bring your arms back so your elbows are pointing to the back, then bring your arms forward and "hug" yourself, your arms crossing in front. Repeat this sequence six times.

TIP:

Keep a diary of when you exercise.
It's a great motivator.

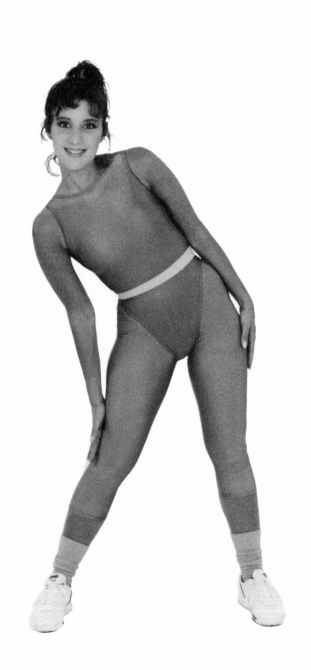

3. Side Bends

Stand comfortably, your arms at your sides, your fingertips touching the outside of your thighs. Slowly bend to the right, at the same time sliding the fingers of your right hand down your right thigh. Do not twist your trunk, and bend only as far as comfortable. Return to starting position, and repeat three times.

Reverse position and bend to the left four times. Repeat entire sequence three times (for a total of twelve bends on each side).

TIP:

Invest in quality shoes; they're better for your feet and will last longer. You don't need to spend a lot of money on attractive exercise clothes—one or two color-coordinated outfits can give a real boost to your self-image.

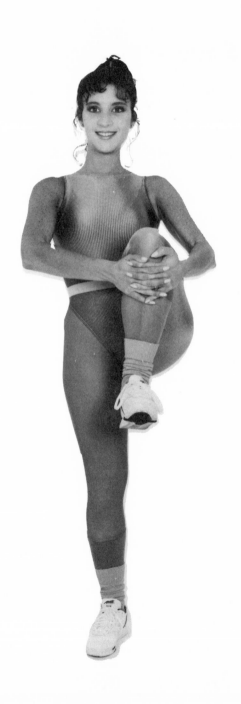

4. Leg Pulls

Stand comfortably, arms at sides. Shift your weight to your left leg and pull your right knee toward your chest with both hands. Pull only as far as you can comfortably manage, and hold a moment, then return to start. Reverse position and pull your left knee toward your chest. Repeat until you have done a total of four pulls with each leg.

TIP:
Work for slow but <u>steady</u> progress. Push yourself to improve week by week but not always day by day.

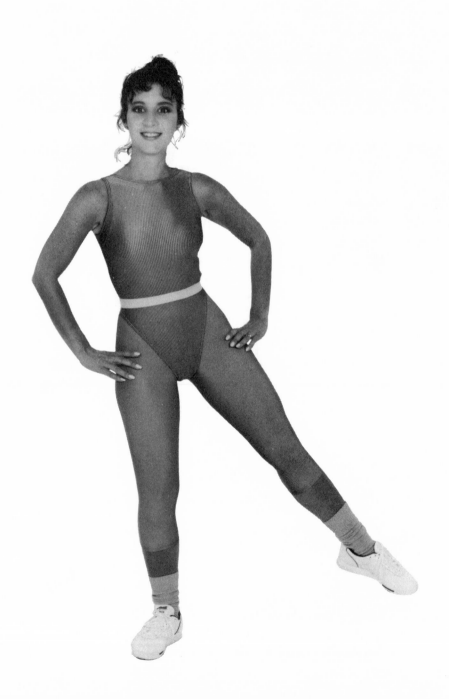

5. Slide Kicks

Stand comfortably with your arms at your sides. Slide your right foot to the right and then up six to eight inches. Lower and repeat. After four slide kicks, repeat on the left side. Repeat entire sequence for a total of eight slide kicks per leg. Keep your standing leg slightly bent each time you kick.

TIP:

Exercising to your favorite music can really enhance your workout; make it a part of your routine.

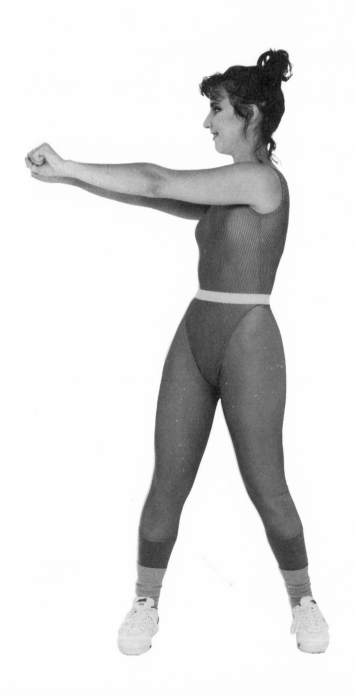

6. Easy Twists

Stand comfortably, your hands out to the front at shoulder level, as if you were holding a broomstick. Twist your arms and torso gently to the right, return to starting position, then twist to the left. Repeat for a total of five twists to each side.

TIP:

Do your workout at least three times a week, but when you get comfortable with this schedule, why not try for five times a week?

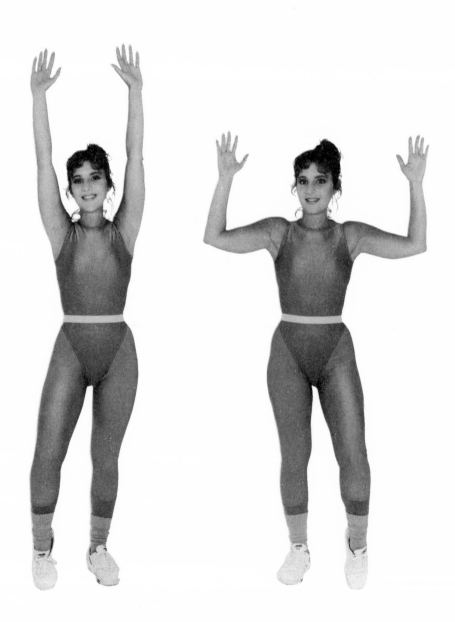

LOW-IMPACT DANCE EXERCISES

1. Walking Tall

Stand comfortably, your feet shoulder-width apart. Keeping the toes of both feet on the floor, raise your right heel. At the same time, stretch both hands high overhead, your palms facing outward.

As you lower your right heel, lift your left heel. At the same time, bend your arms, bringing your upper arms down to shoulder level (as if pulling down a window blind). In effect, you are walking without going anywhere.

Repeat the "steps" and arm movements in a regular rhythm. Start out with as many as you can comfortably do, and work up to forty repetitions (counted by complete sequence of arm movements).

Hint: Start out slowly and gradually increase your pace. As you "walk," keep your stomach sucked in and your rib cage lifted.

Easy alternate: Simply walk in place, using the same arm movements as in the above exercise.

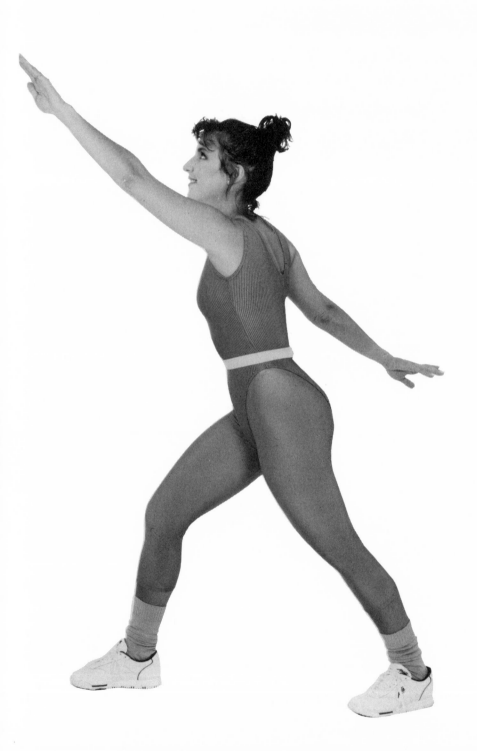

2. Criss Cross

Stand comfortably, feet shoulder-width apart, arms at your sides. On the count of one: *keeping both knees slightly bent, step as far forward as you can with your right foot (your toe is pointed and most of your weight is on your left leg). At the same time, thrust your left arm up and forward, your right arm down and to the back. On the count of* two, *return to starting position.*

On the count of three, *repeat count one, but reverse arm and leg positions. On the count of* four, *return to starting position.*

Start out with as many as you can do comfortably, then work up to twenty repetitions of complete sequence, for a total of forty crosses.

Hint: Don't lean too far forward during counts one and three.

TIP:

Remember to vary your routines. Keep them fresh!

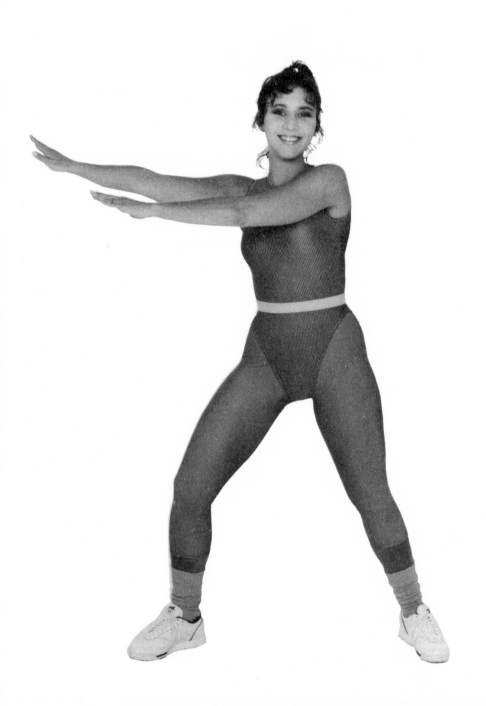

3. Side Slide

Stand with your feet shoulder-width apart. Slightly bending your right leg, the "pivot," turn your trunk to the right and slide your left leg to the side, your toe pointed. At the same time, reach out to the right with both your arms at shoulder level. Return to starting position and repeat, sliding your right leg to the side.

On the count of one, slide left. On count two, slide right.

Start with as many as you can do comfortably and work up to twenty slides on each side.

Hint: The pivot foot shouldn't move as you slide the other foot. Your head should turn toward the sliding foot.

TIP:

Remember always to warm up fully before starting the exercises.

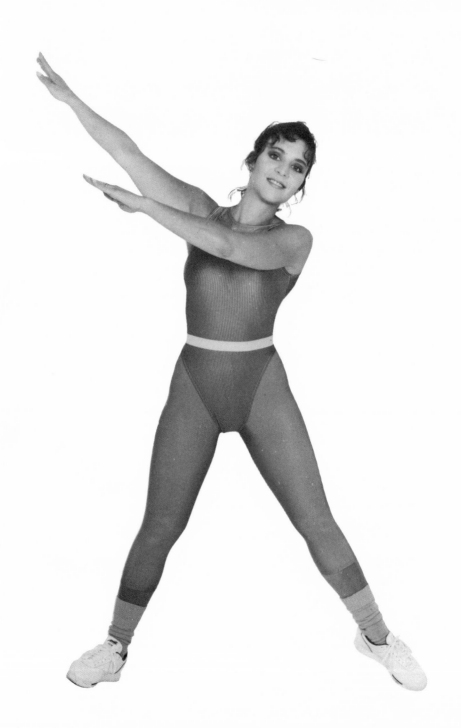

4. Rocking Horse

Stand comfortably, your feet shoulder-width apart. Swing your left leg out to the side. At the same time, reach out and up to the right with both arms. Your trunk should incline slightly to the right.

In a smooth, continuous motion, return your left leg to the floor and swing your right leg out to the right. At the same time, bring your arms down and across your body, then reach up to the left.

Try to develop a smooth, controlled pendulum effect.

Start with four repetitions, and work up to twelve on each side.

TIP:

Working out before your main meal of the day can cut your appetite and help with weight loss.

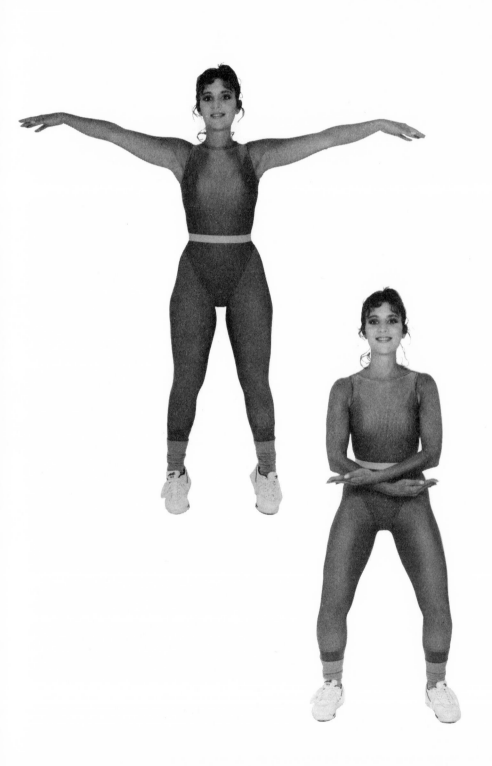

5. Wing Swing

Stand with your feet comfortably apart. On the count of one, rise on your toes and at the same time extend your arms straight out to the sides at shoulder level.

On the count of two, lower your heels to the floor and slightly bend your knees. At the same time, gracefully bring your arms down, crossing your wrists at waist level.

Repeat, aiming for a swinging rhythm of both arms and body.

Hint: Bend your knees only slightly on the downward part of this exercise. Deep knee bends can cause injury.

Easy alternate: If you have difficulty rising on your toes, simply stretch upward on the count of one, reaching as high as you can with your fingertips, feeling a stretching in your torso.

TIP:

Commercial athletic beverages are heavy and sweet; try club soda with a splash of your favorite citrus drink for a great post-exercise thirst quencher.

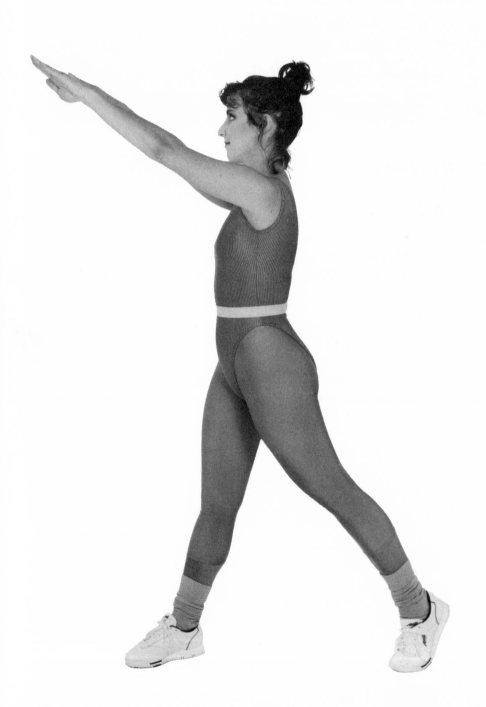

6. Pivot Salute

Stand with your feet shoulder-width apart. On the count of one, twist your upper body to the left and reach upward and out with both arms, feeling the twist throughout your torso. At the same time, point your right foot behind your body.

On the count of two, return to start and gracefully continue through.

On three, repeat step one, on the opposite side.

On four, swing through to start again and continue.

Start with as many as you can do comfortably, and work up to twenty complete cycles.

TIP:

When you travel, don't forget to set aside some time to do your routines. Low-impact aerobics can be done in even the smallest hotel room, and aerobic walking can be a great way to see a new city.

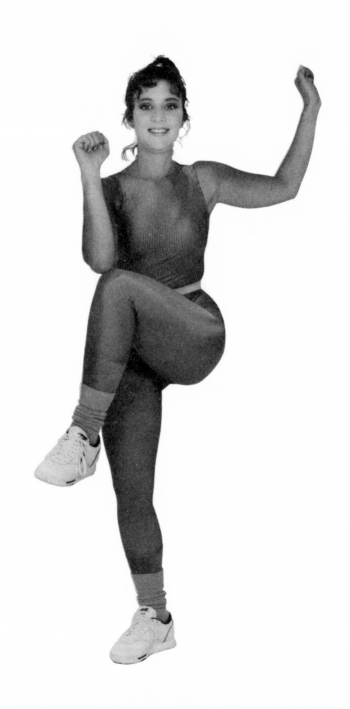

7. Joint Meeting

Stand with your feet shoulder-width apart, arms bent with upper arms parallel to the floor.

On the count of one, lift your left knee as high as you can. At the same time, twist your trunk to the left and bring your right elbow to your knee (or as close to it as you can comfortably manage). On two, return to start.

On three, repeat on the other side, attempting to touch your left elbow to your right knee, and on four return to start.

Repeat in a regular rhythm. Start with as many as you can do comfortably, and work up to twenty repetitions on each side.

TIP:

Some soreness and pain is to be expected, especially when you first start working out. But sharp pain can mean injury. Consult a doctor if you experience severe pain or pain that doesn't go away within a day or two.

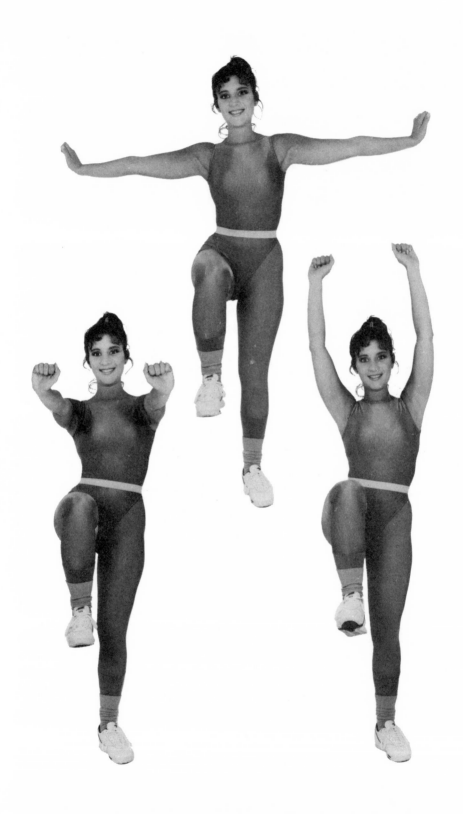

8. Step Up and Punch Out

Stand with your feet shoulder-width apart, arms at sides. March in place, lifting your knees high toward your chest. Each step is one count.

On count one, "punch" both arms straight out in front of you. On two, bring your arms in. Repeat three times (for a total of four).

On three, punch arms straight out to the sides at shoulder level. On four, bring them in. Repeat three times (for a total of four).

On five, punch arms straight up in the air. On six, bring them in. Repeat three times (for a total of four).

On seven, repeat three, and on eight, repeat four.

Start with one complete cycle (four punches each to the front, the sides, up, and to the sides again, for a total of sixteen). Work up to three complete cycles.

If you have not yet worked out for twenty minutes, immediately repeat the entire sequence of exercises. If you have worked out for twenty minutes, move immediately to:

WARMDOWN

Relax your arms and continue marching in place, gradually decreasing the pace.

Stop walking and breathe deeply, in and out. As you do, raise your hands over your head. Lift your left heel off the floor and reach for the ceiling with your right hand. At the same time, inhale deeply. Exhale and relax, then repeat, reaching up with your left hand and raising your right heel. Continue to reach alternately, feeling the stretch throughout your body. After five or six repetitions, sit comfortably on the floor, your legs together and to the front. Reach forward, as far as you can comfortably, and hold your legs for several seconds, feeling the stretch in your torso and thighs.

If you have any favorite relaxing yoga exercises, now is the time to practice them.

Finally, lie on your back, your knees bent, and breathe deeply for two or three minutes.

ALTERNATE EXERCISES

Note: Some of the following exercises are more strenuous than those in the basic routine and should not be attempted by anyone with back or joint trouble.

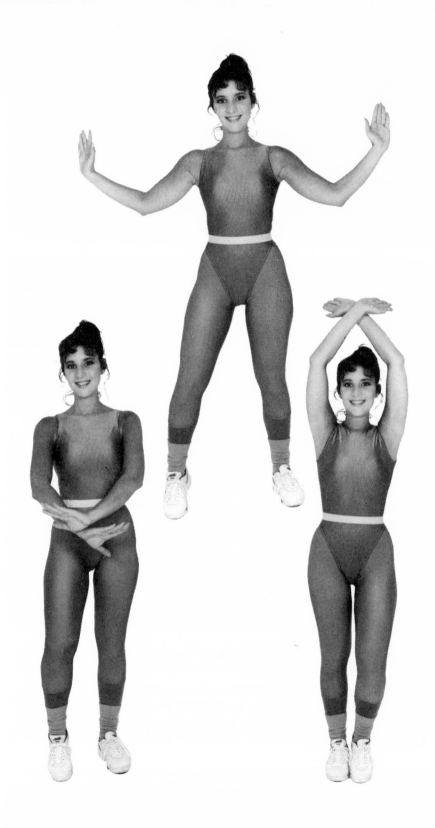

Side Circles

This exercise may be substituted for Exercise #1, or added anywhere in the routine for variety.

Stand comfortably, feet shoulder-width apart, arms relaxed. On the count of one, step to the left with your left foot, followed immediately by your right foot, touching the toe to the floor. At the same time, keeping your arms close to your body and your palms out, make a sweeping outward circle until your hands touch above your head. Imagine that you are washing a very large window.

On the count of two, reverse the foot movements, stepping to the right and circling your arms downward until your hands cross at waist level.

The count should go like this: step-touch circle up; step-touch circle down.

Start with as many as you can do comfortably and work up to thirty on each side.

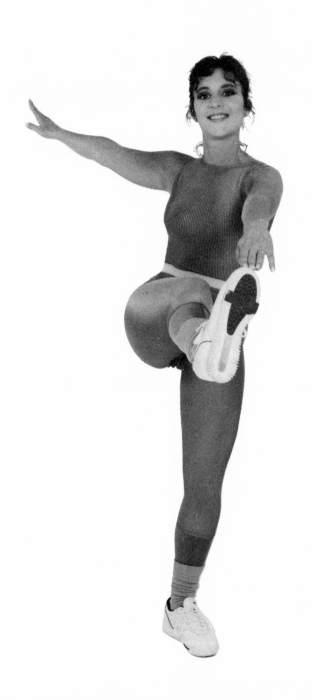

Kick Out

This exercise may be used as an alternate to Exercise #7, or added anywhere for variety. Note that it is somewhat strenuous and should not be attempted if you have back or joint trouble.

Stand with feet shoulder-width apart, knees slightly bent, arms straight out to the sides at shoulder level. On the count of one, kick your left leg out in front. At the same time, without bending your trunk, try to touch your left foot with your right hand.

On the count of two, repeat on the opposite side.

Start out with two on each side, and work up to twelve on each side.

Hint: Always keep the support leg slightly bent when kicking. Kick with control—don't "throw" your leg on the kick. Don't worry about kicking high. Just raise your legs as far as is comfortable.

Dance!

If you like to dance, by all means incorporate your favorite steps into your low-impact dance routine. Remember to work your arms at or above shoulder level while you cha-cha, jitterbug, Charleston, or simply let yourself go with the music.

5

QUESTIONS ABOUT LOW-IMPACT AEROBICS

I've always heard "no pain, no gain." Are low-impact aerobic exercises too easy?

There are two types of pain associated with exercise: the mild pain signaling that your body is being challenged and more severe pain, which can mean injury to a joint or muscle.

When you first begin any exercise program, expect at least some pain as out-of-shape muscles begin to work themselves back into condition. This sort of pain is usually experienced as a mild aching that appears within twelve to thirty-six hours after the unaccustomed activity. The best way to get rid of this sort of pain is to repeat the acitivity that caused it in the first place.

Sudden, acute pain, on the other hand, or a

chronic pain that gets worse during or just after activity, may signal injury, and should be investigated by a doctor.

The notion of "no pain, no gain" comes from the world of competitive weight lifting, where the idea is to overload the muscles with each successive workout, going for the maximum possible effort each time. This philosophy is really suitable only for the most extreme levels of competition; for most people who only wish to get into and stay in shape, a more gentle level of exercise is all that is necessary. However, it is possible that for some people low-impact aerobics is indeed too "easy"; see the following, related question.

I can't get my pulse rate into my target zone. What am I doing wrong?

If you are following the instructions and exercising vigorously for twenty minutes, the chances are you are doing nothing wrong. Rather, your own aerobic capacity is already good, and the workouts are not quite vigorous enough to challenge you.

Check to make sure you are doing the routines correctly. Have someone watch as you work out to make sure that you are continuously exercising for twenty minutes. During your walk, monitor yourself. Are you stopping to window shop? Do you slow down to a stroll without thinking about it?

If you are certain that you are exercising correctly, then you need to increase the challenge of the exercise. The first thing to try is working at a faster pace: walk faster and try to perform the dance routines more quickly. You can also try doing the dance routines with wrist weights, which increase the difficulty of the workout. Do not use weights heavier than one pound (you can simply hold one-pound cans in your hands), and do not use ankle weights, which can damage your joints. Also, don't use any sort of weights in your walking program.

Finally, if nothing else helps, consider switching to a more strenuous aerobic activity such as race-walking, swimming, or jogging.

Should I work out if I'm sick?

The answer to this question depends partly on what you mean by "sick." If you feel so awful that you can hardly get out of bed, you certainly shouldn't consider exercising. Likewise, if you're running a fever, stay quiet, drink plenty of fluids, and postpone your aerobic workout to another day.

If you just have a slight case of sniffles, however, or are feeling generally "blah," by all means do your regular workout. You will probably find, as do most regular exercisers, that the activity will make you feel better, physically and mentally.

What about aerobics classes?

Doing low-impact aerobics in a class is an excellent idea for several reasons. Not only is it easier for most people to exercise as part of a group, the routines are easier to follow with an instructor to model the steps for you. In fact, familiarity with a class routine may make it easier for you to work out on your own at home. Be certain that any class you attend is taught by an experienced instructor who is familiar with the principles of low-impact aerobic exercise.

If you cannot find a convenient low-impact aerobics class, it's almost as good to rent a videotaped workout and follow it on your VCR. Try several tapes until you find one or two that you enjoy.

Even if you don't go to a class or follow a tape on a regular basis, doing so occasionally can provide a real lift, helping you to keep your routines fresh and interesting.

ACKNOWLEDGMENTS

I want to thank the following people for help in preparing this book: Maria Agardy, for her moral support and advice on warmup exercises; Dr. Steven Blair of the Institute for Aerobics Research, for his expertise and advice on all aspects of aerobics; Dorrie Anthony, for her friendship and support throughout this project; Debbie Rubin, for her knowledgeable feedback and modeling services; and finally, Jill LeVine for her patience, tact, exceptional good humor, and skill as a photographer.